Heart Sounds

Heart Sounds

A Cardiac Auscultation Primer

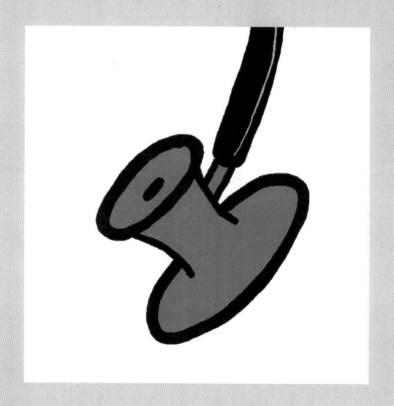

Christopher Hanifin

ISBN 1452840059
LCCN 2010907491

Hanifin, Christopher
  Heart sounds: a cardiac auscultation primer / Christopher Hanifin
      p.;cm.
  Includes index.
  ISBN 1452840055 (pbk.)
  1. Cardiology—Handbooks, manuals, etc. 2. Physical Diagnosis–
Handbooks, manuals, etc.
  [DNLM: 1. Cardiac Diseases– Handbooks.]

Medicine is a rapidly changing science. Care has been taken to confirm
the accuracy of the information presented in this book and to outline basic,
general principles. However the author and publishers are not responsible
for any errors or omissions or for any consequences related to the applica-
tion of the information in this book and make no warranty, express or im-
plied, with respect to the contents of this publication. It is the responsibil-
ity of the practitioner, relying on experience and knowledge of the patient,
to determine the appropriate diagnosis and treatment .

To order additional copies of this book, please visit:
http://tinyurl.com/HeartSoundsBook

This book is dedicated to the ladies in my life:
Debra and Abigail.

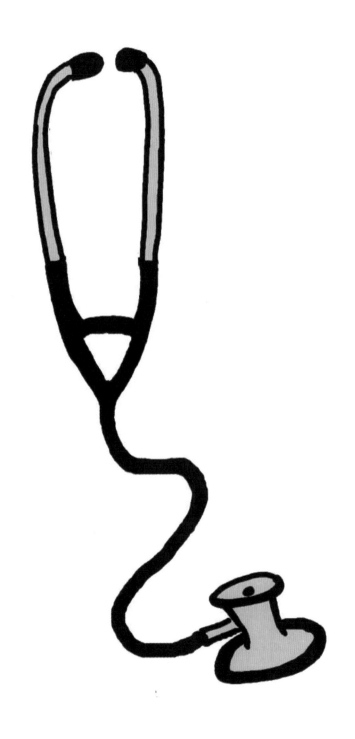

Contents

Acknowledgements

Like many books, this one was on the mind for a long time before making its way onto paper. It never would have done so without the generous support and encouragement of my colleagues at Seton Hall.

Thanks to the many students with whom I have crossed paths through the years. Your curiosity and insight have continuously challenged me and encouraged this work.

Thanks to the many excellent clinicians that I have had the opportunity to work with and learn from. The first physicians I had contact with were, naturally, my personal physicians. John Butler, MD and E. Allen Speidell, MD both provided calm, compassionate care with a good sense of humor and good, old-fashioned common sense. The skilled hands of the surgeons at Cardiothoracic Surgery of South Bend taught me a great deal. Particular thanks go to Walter Halloran, MD who excelled as a teacher, mentor and all-around good guy. Thanks to William Min, MD for demonstrating a legendary work ethic and to Kevin Gillespie, MD for serving as a constant reminder that medicine has a lighter side.

And finally, no thanks are complete without acknowledging my family, especially my parents John and Mary. Words cannot properly express the thanks that would be needed for years of unwavering support in all my endeavors. If I live to be half the person my parents are, I will consider my life well-lived.

Introduction

The stethoscope has long been a symbol of medical practice, but clinicians beginning their career quickly discover that proficiency with a stethoscope is a hard-earned skill. Given the easy availability of technology (particularly echocardiography), many clinicians may have the impression that cardiac auscultation is not a cost-effective skill to learn in terms of the time investment required to develop expertise.

Cardiac auscultation may be complex in some situations, but all clinicians should possess a basic level of competence. Reviewing cardiac auscultation in a physical examination textbook may make the task seem especially daunting as the reader is presented with tables that may be very difficult to memorize. This book takes another approach: systematically using knowledge you already possess from anatomy and physiology classes to assist you in diagnosing the vast majority of abnormal heart sounds.

This book takes the form of a programmed text. Programmed texts have demonstrated success in teaching a variety of concepts in medicine such as ECG interpretation, chest radiograph interpretation and the neurologic examination. This book also assumes that the reader has had instruction in the fundamentals of cardiac anatomy and physiology.

Each page presents one or two key concepts using a few sentences and a simple sketch or two. The reader is then invited to answer some questions to ensure that the concepts on each page have been understood. Repetition is used to reinforce concepts. By linking simple concepts together and building upon them, the reader will develop a foundation for understanding cardiac auscultation.

There is no audio material associated with this book. The reader can find many high-quality recordings available from a variety of sources for further study and practice. Without a solid understanding of the concepts presented in a book like this, even the best recordings may only add to a novice's confusion. If you listen to a chest or recording and hear:

"LUB DaDUP"

and cannot decide if it is a split S2 or an S3, this book is for you.

This book is intended to present a fundamental understanding of cardiac auscultation for students of medicine, allied health and nursing. It is by no means sufficient in itself. There is no substitute for time in the clinic. So after reading, hit the wards and happy listening!

A Touch of Physics

Remember all those hours in physics class spent wondering, "When will I ever have use for this information again?" (If the subject was electromagnetism, the answer may well be "never.")

Physics may not be far behind organic chemistry in terms of its ability to provoke dread among premedical students. Have no fear, proficiency at cardiac auscultation will not require you to recall all those equations that once kept you up late into the night.

However, a very brief review of some basic principles related to fluid movement and sound conduction will assist in understanding heart sounds.

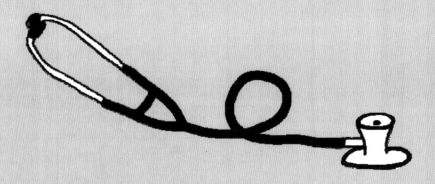

Key Points:

Blood flow is regulated by physics principles that you are already familiar with.

- Like all fluids, blood flows from an area of high pressure to an area of low pressure.

- Valves open and close in response to pressure differences (gradients) on either side of the valve.

- If a defect in the circulatory system allows communication between the systemic and pulmonary circulation, blood usually flows from the systemic (left side) to the pulmonary (right side) circulation.

- Laminar flow is generally quiet. Turbulent flow generates sound.

Pressure

Like all fluids, blood will flow from an area of high pressure to an area of low pressure. In general, the higher the **pressure gradient**, the higher the velocity of flow. The unit of measurement that will be used for pressure in this book is millimeters of mercury (mmHg.) This unit should be familiar - it is used in blood pressure measurement.

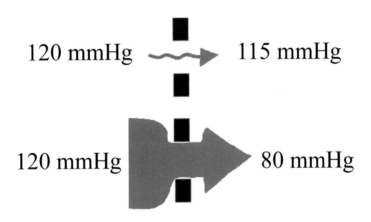

120 mmHg ⟶ 115 mmHg

120 mmHg ⟶ 80 mmHg

Higher gradient = Higher flow

Blood flow (like all fluid movement) is controlled by _____. Fluid moves from an area of ____ pressure to an area of _____ pressure. As the pressure difference between two areas increases, the _____ of blood flow increases.	Pressure gradients High, Low Velocity

Pressure

Since valves are subject to the laws of physics, they open and close according to these laws. Thus, valve opening and closing is determined by pressure gradients. The images below demonstrate that a valve normally opens when the pressure behind it exceeds the pressure in front of it.

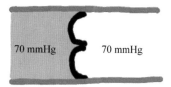

In this illustration, no pressure gradient exists across the valve, so no flow is taking place.

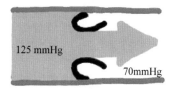

Pressure behind the valve now exceeds pressure in front of it. This 55mmHg gradient has caused the valve to open, and blood is ejected.

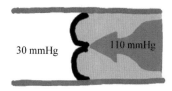

Pressure in front of the valve now exceeds pressure behind it. The valve has been pushed closed to prevent retrograde blood flow.

_____ determine when heart valves will open and when they will close.

A properly functioning valve will ____ when the pressure behind it exceeds the pressure in front of it.

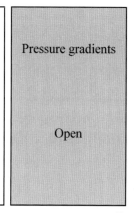

Pressure gradients

Open

Pressure

Blood will also flow down a pressure gradient through any abnormal connection present in heart or in the circulatory system. Under normal circumstances the gradient will cause blood to flow from the systemic circulation to the pulmonary circulation.

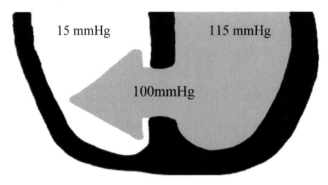

15 mmHg   115 mmHg

100mmHg

In the picture above, there is a defect in the septum. A 100mmHg pressure gradient exists between the high-pressure left ventricle (gray) to the low-pressure right ventricle (white). This gradient causes blood to flow from the left ventricle into right ventricle as illustrated.

If an abnormal connection exists between the systemic and pulmonic circulation, blood will flow down a _____ if one exists.

In the absence of other pathology, this flow is usually from the _____ circulation to the _____ circulation.

Pressure gradient

Systemic, Pulmonic

Turbulence

Smooth fluid flow through a vessel is referred to as **"laminar"** flow. Friction between the fluid and vessel wall slows the edge of the fluid column, but the flow remains orderly. Laminar flow is usually silent.

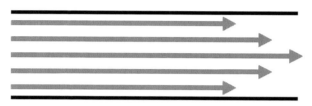

When laminar flow is interrupted by an obstruction, turbulence develops. If the degree of turbulence becomes increasingly severe it will eventually produce sound: Turbulent Flow = Noise

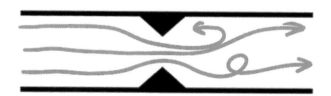

Smooth, _____ flow is generally silent.	Laminar
Obstructions lead to turbulence which produces _____ .	Sound
You use this principle to measure blood pressure. Inflating the cuff obstructs an artery producing _____ sounds.	Korotkoff

Sound Conduction

Fluid is a fairly efficient carrier of sound. As a result, murmurs generally **radiate** to predictable locations. For example, a murmur which is heard over an abnormality...

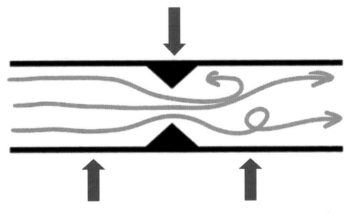

...will also often be heard **proximal** and **distal** to the abnormality. (Depending upon the degree of turbulence present.)

A murmur may be heard directly over an abnormal area, but it will also often be heard _____ and _____ to the abnormality.	Proximal, Distal
Therefore, to diagnose a murmur, it is important to consider the _____ of blood flow involved. (Knowledge of anatomy is important!)	Direction

Sound Conduction

Applying the information on the previous page, we can recognize that murmurs associated with pathology in a particular valve tend to travel to predictable locations.

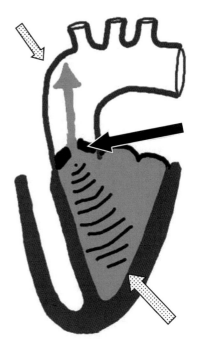

In the example pictured here, the aortic valve is narrowed causing a murmur over the valve (black arrow). A jet of blood is projected into the aorta producing a murmur there (upper arrow). Finally, some sound may also be transmitted through the blood itself backward into the left ventricle (lower arrow).

Murmurs often transmit sounds or ____ to predictable locations.

For example, a murmur heard over the aorta and the left ventricle suggests pathology in the ____ valve, which lies between these structures.

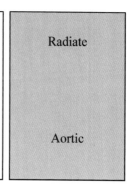

Radiate

Aortic

Cardiac Anatomy

Considering the amount of work that the heart performs over the course of a lifetime, cardiac anatomy is fairly simple. The heart is a two-sided pump which will contract approximately two billion times in the course of an average lifespan.

Before becoming overwhelmed with the potential complexity of heart sounds, consider that there are only four valves. Knowledge about where these valves are located and the direction which blood usually passes through them is essential in diagnosing a murmur (and greatly reduces the need to memorize things!)

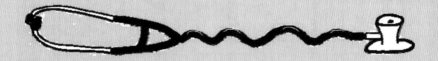

Key Points:

- The heart is a two-sided pump.
    - The right side of the heart pumps into the pulmonary circulation and is a low-pressure system.
    - The left side of the heart pumps into the systemic circulation and operates under much higher pressures.

- The heart is somewhat rotated in the chest. This rotation causes much of the left ventricle to lie posterior to the right ventricle.

- The cardiac "apex" lies inferior to the cardiac "base."

- Four major valves are present in the heart to promote unidirectional flow through its chambers.
    - Atrioventricular valves lie between the atria and ventricles.
    - Semilunar valves lie between the ventricles and the great vessels.

Surface Anatomy

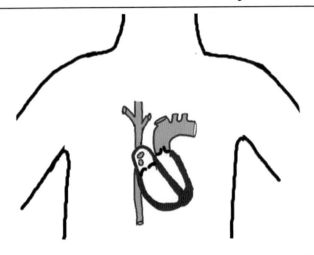

The heart is a four-chambered organ consisting of two pumps. The right chambers function as a low-pressure pump sending blood into the pulmonary circulation. The high-pressure left side pumps into the systemic circulation.

The heart sits slightly rotated in the chest. Because of this, most of the left ventricle is posterior to the right ventricle. The tip (apex) of the left ventricle usually lies at the fifth intercostal space medial to the left mid-clavicular line.

The cardiac apex generally lies at the _____ interspace.

While we have "right" and "left" ventricles, the heart is rotated in the chest with much of the left ventricle _____ to the right ventricle.

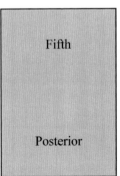

Fifth

Posterior

Transverse View

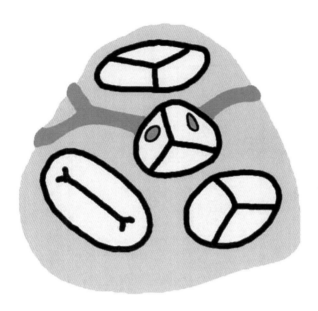

The heart is often depicted with the aortic and pulmonic valves superior to the mitral and tricuspid valves. In reality, all of the valves lie in a plane in a band of fibrous tissue in the center of the heart.

The valve at the center of the picture above is the _____ valve. (Hint: Those gray structures are coronary arteries.)	Aortic
The valve in the lower left of the picture is the _____ valve. (Hint: How many leaflets are there?)	Mitral (or bicuspid)

Right Ventricle

The right ventricle operates under fairly low pressure. Venous blood from the body enters the right ventricle through the **tricuspid valve**. During systole, blood exits the ventricle through the **pulmonic valve**.

Since the right ventricle receives blood from the body, problems in the right ventricle – whether due to valvular problems or other pathology - will often cause blood to "back up" into the venous system.

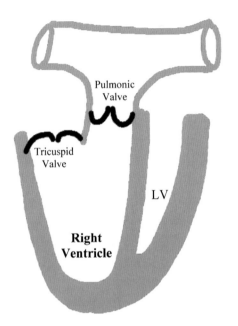

Right ventricle demonstrating the locations of the tricuspid and pulmonic valves.

The right side of the heart is a _____ pressure system.	Low
The right ventricle receives blood from the vena cavae and pumps into the _____ circulation.	Pulmonary
Two valves control blood flow through the right ventricle: blood enters through the _____ valve and exits through the _____ valve.	Tricuspid, Pulmonic

Left Ventricle

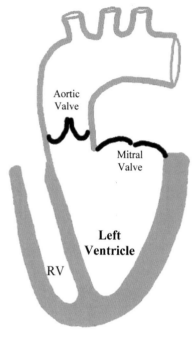

Left ventricle demonstrating the locations of the mitral and aortic valves.

The left ventricle is the workhorse of the heart, pumping into the high-pressure systemic circulation. It is more muscular and thicker than the right ventricle. Blood enters the left ventricle through the **mitral valve** and exits through the **aortic valve**.

Anatomically, much of the left ventricle lies tucked behind the right ventricle which can make auscultation of the left ventricle a little tricky...

The left ventricle pumps into the _____ circulation.	Systemic
The left side of the heart is a _____ pressure system.	High
Two valves control blood flow through the left ventricle: the _____ valve and the _____ valve.	Mitral (or bicuspid), Aortic

Atrioventricular (AV) Valves

As the name suggests, the **atrioventricular (AV) valves** lie between the atria and ventricles. They depend upon fairly complex anchoring apparatus (the **papillary muscles** and **chordae tendinae**) to function properly.

It is also noteworthy that the AV valves depend upon proper ventricular wall function to operate properly.

The **tricuspid valve** is located on the right side of the heart and the **mitral valve** is located on the left side of the heart.

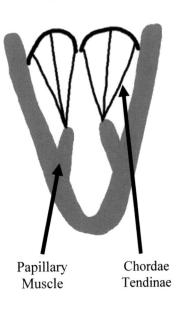

Papillary
Muscle

Chordae
Tendinae

The atrioventricular valves separate the atria from the ventricles. They are the _____ valve and the _____ valve.	Mitral, Tricuspid
The structure of the AV valves is complex. They are connected to anchoring apparatus called the _____ and the_____.	Papillary muscles, Chordae tendinae
AV vales depend upon proper ventricular contraction to close properly. Conditions like _____ may make the ventricular wall stiff and cause valve dysfunction.	Myocardial ischemia

Semilunar Valves

The structure of the **semilunar valves** is somewhat less complex than the structure of the AV valves. The semilunar valves are composed of three deep cusps which present a large surface area for meeting.

Blood traverses the semilunar valves when it exits the ventricles and enters the great vessels. The **pulmonic valve** lies at the exit of the right ventricle. The **aortic valve** lies at the exit of the left ventricle.

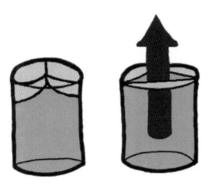

The semilunar valves are located at the junction of the heart with the _____ and _____.	Aorta, Pulmonary artery
The semilunar valves are the _____ and _____ valves.	Aortic, Pulmonic
The structure of the semilunar valves is a little less complex than the structure of the AV valves. They lack anchoring apparatus and are composed of three deep _____ .	Cusps (or leaflets)

The Cardiac Cycle

It is impossible to intelligently assess heart sounds without an adequate understanding of the cardiac cycle. Knowing which valves should normally be open or closed during both systole and diastole is essential to developing a differential diagnosis for abnormal heart sounds. In a tachycardiac patient, it is also sometimes surprisingly difficult to distinguish systole from diastole.

The examples which follow will primarily consider left side of the heart. The left side of the heart operates under higher pressure and makes a more significant contribution to the sounds heard during cardiac auscultation.

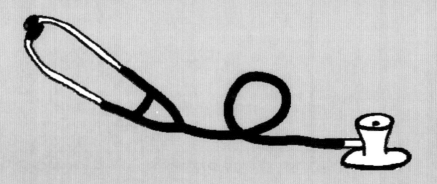

Key Points:

- During diastole, the atrioventricular valves open allowing blood to fill the ventricles.

- As systole begins, the atrioventricular valves close producing the heart sound called S1.

- As systole continues, the semilunar valves open, allowing blood to travel from the ventricles into the great vessels.

- When systole ends, the semilunar valves close, producing the heart sound called S2.

- The valves on the left side of the heart function under higher pressure and therefore produce louder sounds than the valves on the right side of the heart.

Diastole

Diastole is the resting phase of the cardiac cycle. During diastole, the ventricles normally fill through wide-open atrioventricular valves.

Since healthy valves do not usually produce a murmur, *diastole is silent in the absence of pathology*.

Diastole concludes with atrial systole (contraction), when the atria contract to complete filling of the ventricles.

At resting heart rates, diastole is usually noticeably longer than systole.

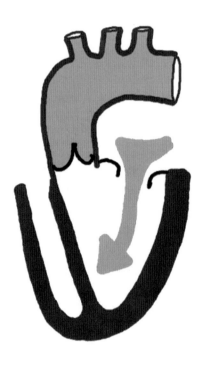

During diastole, the heart is filling in preparation for the next contraction (also called _____).	Systole
During diastole, the _____ valves are usually open and the _____ valves are usually closed.	AV, Semilunar
In the absence of pathology, diastole is _____.	Silent

Early Systole: S1

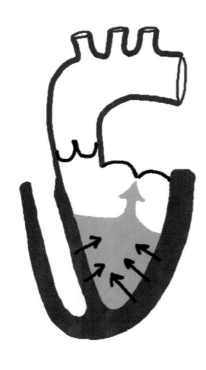

As **systole** (ventricular contraction) begins, intraventricular pressure rapidly rises. Blood pushes against the atrioventricular valves causing them to close. This produces the heart sound called S1.

The ventricles continue to contract while both the AV and semilunar valves remain closed. This period is referred to as isovolumetric contraction.

Finally, when intraventricular pressure exceeds the pressure in the great vessels, the semilunar valves open.

When ventricular systole begins, pressure within the ventricles rapidly _____.	Increases
When intraventricular pressure rises above atrial pressure, the _____ valve and the _____ valve will close.	Tricuspid, Mitral
In the absence of pathology, these two valves close simultaneously producing the heart sound called _____.	S1

Mid Systole: Ejection

As systole continues, intra-ventricular pressure eventually surpasses the pressure in the great vessels. When this occurs, the semilunar valves open.

In the example pictured here, pressure in the left ventricle has risen above aortic pressure. The aortic valve has opened and blood is being ejected into the aorta.

The right ventricle is simultaneously pumping blood into the pulmonary artery.

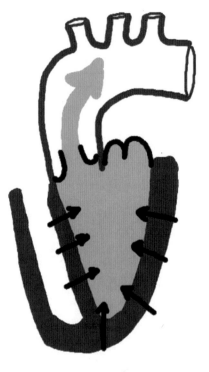

As intraventricular pressure rises, it eventually surpasses pressure in the great vessels. This pressure increase causes the _____ valve and the _____ valve to open.	Aortic, Pulmonic
A healthy valve presents little resistance to flow. In the absence of pathology, ejection of blood through these valves is generally _____.	Silent
The aortic valve remains open as long as pressure in the _____ is higher than pressure in the _____.	Left Ventricle Aorta

End Systole: S2

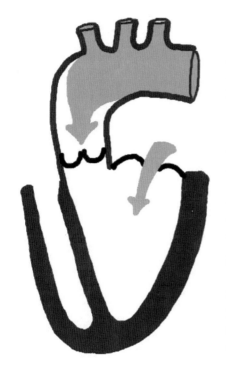

As systole concludes, intra-ventricular pressure rapidly drops. When the pressure in the ventricles drops below the pressure in the great vessels, the semilunar valves close.

In the example pictured, left ventricular pressure has dropped below aortic pressure. As blood attempts to flow backward into the ventricle, the aortic valve closes. The mitral valve opens and a new cycle begins.

Similar events occur with the pulmonic valve and the tricuspid valve on the right side of the heart.

As systole ends, pressure in the ventricles drops below the pressure in the great vessels. This leads to closure of the _____ valve and the _____ valve.

Aortic, Pulmonic

The closure of these two valves produces the heart sound called _____. (Sometimes these valves do not close simultaneously. This situation causes "splitting" of S2—more on this later...)

S2

The _____ valves open and the ventricles begin to fill with blood, beginning a new cycle.

Atrioventricular

The Cardiac Examination

A thoughtful examination of the cardiovascular system requires two things which are unfortunately often in short supply in a medical environment: time and a quiet room.

Clinicians should recognize that a cursory cardiac examination may miss subtle but significant findings indicative of serious pathology.

While this book is devoted to cardiac auscultation, it must be recognized that auscultation should take place within the context of a complete history and physical examination. Inspection and palpation are essential in developing a differential diagnosis for abnormal heart sounds.

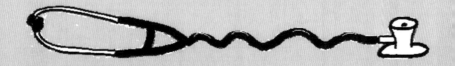

Key Points:

- Cardiac auscultation is only one component of the cardiac physical examination.

- Inspection (particularly of the neck vessels) can often provide very useful insight into cardiac function.

- When a murmur is discovered, palpation is a necessary component of assessment.

- Cardiac auscultation requires a careful assessment of both high-pitched and low-pitched sounds.

Inspection

In a modern healthcare system, it would be unusual for a patient to develop pathology significant enough to produce visual findings on the chest wall, but lifts and heaves remain possible. These findings represent significant pathologic enlargement of one or more cardiac chambers.

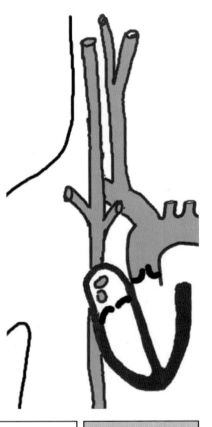

Careful **inspection** for subtle findings may still yield much useful information. Inspection of the neck vessels in particular is important due to their intimate relationship with the heart. When the tricuspid valve is open, pressure in the jugular veins approximates pressure in the right ventricle.

Examination of the jugular veins can provide insight into _____ heart function.	Right
For example, regurgitation through the _____ valve might allow blood to flow into the superior vena cava with each systole.	Tricuspid

Palpation

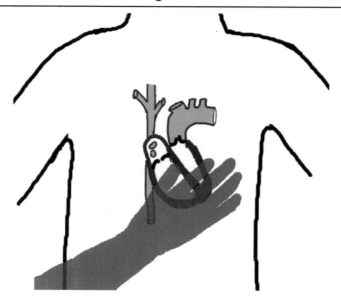

Palpation is an important component of the cardiac examination, and is essential in a patient with a murmur. Blood flow which has become extremely turbulent can produce a palpable vibration called a **"thrill"** - such a vibration indicates a pathologic condition. Palpation also helps to precisely locate the cardiac apex where the left ventricle is heard best.

Palpation helps to locate the cardiac _____ where sounds from the left ventricle are best heard.	Apex
If a murmur is associated with a palpable vibration called a _____, a pathologic condition should be suspected.	Thrill

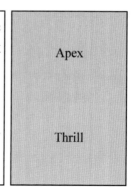

Auscultation

Most traditional stethoscopes have two sides: a **bell** and a **diaphragm**. To switch between using the bell and diaphragm, the head of the stethoscope is rotated on its tubing. Some newer stethoscopes feature a single head with a "floating diaphragm" design which combines the functions of a bell and diaphragm.

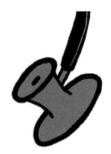

Proper cardiac auscultation demands a search for low-pitched sounds. Failure to listen for low-pitched sounds may cause a clinician to overlook significant pathology. To hear low-pitched sounds, the bell (or floating diaphragm) must be applied to the skin very lightly. Applying firm pressure stretches the skin and may block the transmission of low-pitched sounds.

Remember: low sounds = low pressure.

Bonus question: The first stethoscope was invented in France in 1816 by _____ _____.	Rene Laennec
The two sides of a stethoscope head are designed to listen for different sounds. The bell is used to listen for ___ sounds, while the diaphragm is used to listen for ___ sounds.	Low-pitched, High-pitched
To work properly, the bell must be applied directly to the skin with _____ pressure.	Light

Auscultation Locations

At a minimum, cardiac auscultation is usually performed at the areas indicated below. It is worth noting that the named areas do not always overlie the valve they are named for. For example, the "aortic area" does not overlie the aortic valve.

Aortic Area (right second interspace): This site does not overlie the aortic valve, but the area where some sounds related to aortic valve pathology are likely to be projected.

Pulmonic Area (left second interspace): This site does not overlie the pulmonic valve, but the area where sounds related to pulmonic valve pathology are likely to be projected.

Erb's Point (left third interspace): This site is in close proximity to the semilunar valves. S2 is heard well at this location.

Tricuspid Area (left fourth/fifth interspaces at the sternal border): This site overlies the right ventricle.

Mitral Area (cardiac apex, usually in the fifth interspace): This location "hears" the left ventricle best.

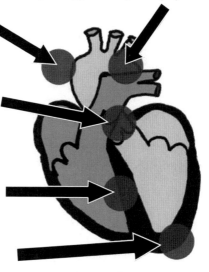

Although most auscultation areas are named after valves, they do not necessarily overlie a valve. Instead, they overlie the location where sounds from valve pathology are often _____.

To properly identify the mitral area, a clinician should ____ the apical impulse.

Projected

Palpate

Heart Sounds

This chapter discusses the origins of normal and abnormal heart sounds.

When one considers abnormal cardiac auscultory findings the first thing that likely comes to mind are murmurs. In addition to heart murmurs, there is another family of abnormal auscultory findings: added (or extra) heart sounds. Whereas a murmur is a continuous sound occurring during blood flow, added sounds are usually discreet "snaps," "pops" and "clicks" that are related to conditions such as stiffened myocardium or stenotic valves popping open. Added heart sounds may be associated with a heart murmur or they may occur independently.

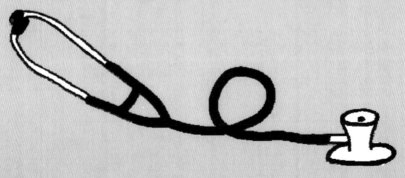

Key Points:

- The first sound, S1, occurs with AV valve closure and marks the beginning of systole.

- The second sound, S2 occurs with semilunar valve closure and marks the beginning of diastole.

- If valves on the left and right sides of the heart fail to close simultaneously, splitting of S1 or S2 will result.

- Splitting of S1 represents a pathologic condition

- Splitting of S2 during inspiration is often a normal finding. Fixed splitting of S2 is classically associated with an atrial septal defect.

- The appearance of an S3 or an S4 usually indicates that the heart is stressed.

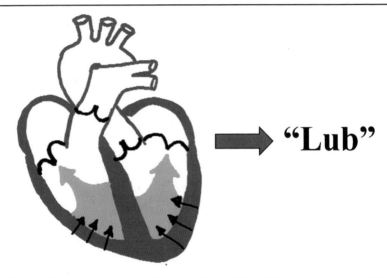

The first heart sound is called "**S1.**" It is produced by closure of the atrioventricular valves. S1 marks the beginning of systole. S1 is loudest at the apex, which may help to distinguish S1 from S2 in a tachycardic patient.

S1 is commonly referred to as a "**LUB**" sound.

S1 represents closure of the _____ valves.	Atrioventricular
S1 marks the beginning of _____.	Systole
S1 is loudest at the _____.	Apex
S1 produces a sound that sounds like _____.	LUB

The first heart sound is actually the fusion of two sounds, "**M1**" and "**T1**." M1 is the sound produced by the closure of the mitral valve and T1 is the sound produced by closure of the tricuspid valve. M1 is usually louder than T1.

These valves normally close almost simultaneously, so usually only one sound is perceived. Failure of the valves to close simultaneously may produce two distinct sounds. This is referred to as "splitting."

S1 ("LUB") = simultaneous M1 + T1

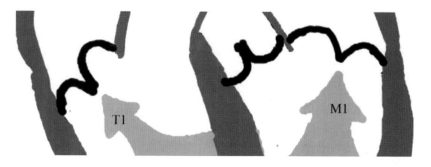

The two components of S1 are _____ and _____.	M1 (Mitral), T1 (Tricuspid)
These valves usually close _____.	Simultaneously
If the valves fail to close synchronously, _____ may be heard.	Splitting
_____ is normally a louder sound than ____.	M1, T1

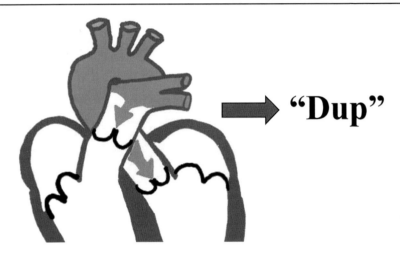

"Dup"

The second heart sound is called "**S2**." It is produced by closure of the semilunar valves. S2 is loudest directly over the valves at the left third intercostal space. S2 marks the beginning of diastole.

S2 is commonly referred to as a "DUP" sound.

S2 represents closure of the _____ valves.	Semilunar
S2 marks the beginning of _____.	Diastole
S2 is loudest at the _____.	Left third intercostal space
S2 produces a sounds that sounds like _____.	DUP

S2

S2 is also composed of two sounds, aortic valve closure (**A2**) and pulmonic valve closure (**P2**). A2 is normally louder than P2.

Breathing causes hemodynamic changes and influences the timing of these sounds. Inspiration frequently causes A2 to precede P2, resulting in splitting. This finding is normal.

S2 ("DUP") = simultaneous A2 + P2

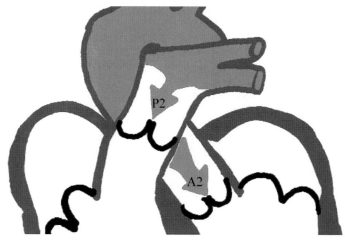

The two components of S2 are _____ and _____.	A2, P2
_____ is usually the louder component of S2.	A2
These sounds may normally split during _____.	Inspiration

Splitting of Heart Sounds

Normally, the AV valves close synchronously and the semilunar valves close synchronously, producing single sounds. If the right-sided and left-sided valves close significantly out of sync, an extra sound will become apparent.

If S1 sounds like "LUB," splitting of S1 adds an extra syllable to produce a new sound: "**laLUB**."
- As an example, if the mitral valve closes before the tricuspid valve, M1 will be heard as "la" and T1 will become "LUB" → laLUB DUP... laLUB DUP...

S2 sounds like "DUP." Splitting of S2 adds an extra syllable, producing "**daDUP**."
- As another example, if the aortic valve has closed before the pulmonic valve, A2 produces the "da" sound and P2 becomes "DUP" → LUB daDUP... LUB daDUP...

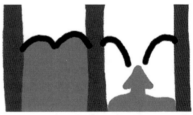

This image depicts two valves that should normally close synchronously, producing a single sound. In this case, one has closed before the other. Splitting will result.

When valves do not close synchronously, the result is _____ of heart sounds.	Splitting
Splitting of S1 is always _____.	Pathologic
Splitting of S2 is sometimes _____.	Normal

Split S1

As previously noted, the atrioventricular valves normally close synchronously in response to simultaneous contraction of the ventricles. For S1 to be split either:

- the ventricles contract out of synchrony

or

- there is a disturbance in the normal pressure in the systemic or pulmonary circuit.

A noticeable split of S1 indicates the presence of a pathologic condition.

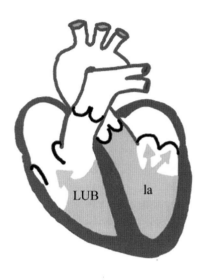

In this illustration, the mitral valve has closed before the tricuspid valve. The first heart sound now has two syllables:

laLUB DUP... laLUB DUP...

S1 represents closure of the _____ valves.	Atrioventricular
Splitting of S1 is _____.	Pathologic
Splitting of S1 means either the ventricles _____ out of sync, or there is a _____ disturbance in the systemic or pulmonic circulation.	Contract, Pressure

Split S2

Assessing a split S2 is a little more complex than assessing a split S1:

- **Inspiratory splitting** of S2 is a normal response to hemodynamic changes. During inspiration, intra-thoracic pressure drops, increasing venous return to the heart.
- **Fixed splitting** which does not disappear with exhalation is pathologic and *usually indicative of an atrial septal defect*.
- **Reverse or paradoxical splitting of S2** - splitting with exhalation - also indicates a pathologic condition.

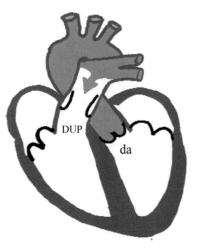

In this image, the aortic valve has closed while the pulmonic valve is still open. This asynchrony will lead to a split S2:

LUB daDUP... LUB daDUP...

S2 represents closure of the _____ valves.

Splitting of S2 may occur in normal subjects during _____.

Fixed splitting of S2 usually represents an _____.

Semilunar

Inspiration

Atrial septal defect

S3

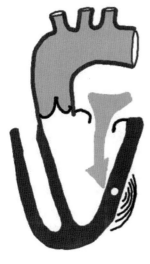

An "**S3**" is an added heart sound. It occurs early in diastole, immediately after S2. S3 is also sometimes referred to as a "ventricular gallop."

In asymptomatic patients under age 30, an S3 is considered a benign finding. Over the age of 30, an S3 is generally considered an indicator of a stressed heart. It is thought to represent blood flowing into a stiff ventricle.

Due to the fact that it is usually very low-pitched, an S3 may be missed unless auscultation is performed with the bell of the stethoscope.

As a mnemonic, some clinicians say that the cadence of an S1-S2+S3 sounds like the cadence of the word "Kentucky" with:

"Ken" = S1   "tuc" = S2   "ky" = S3.

An S3 is a sound which immediately follows ____.	S2
S3 is usually a very ___ pitched sound.	Low
S3 is believed to indicate that a condition like ischemia or heart failure has caused the ventricle to become _____.	Stiff

S4

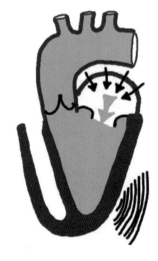

An "**S4**" is another added heart sound which usually indicates a stressed heart. S4 is sometimes referred to as an "atrial gallop." It occurs late in diastole just before S1. It is believed to represent atrial contraction pushing blood into a stiff ventricle.

Like S3, S4 is also usually a low-pitched sound best heard with the bell of the stethoscope.

Some clinicians say that the cadence of an S4+S1 S2 resembles the cadence of the word "Tennessee" with:

"Ten" = S4 "nes" = S1   "see" = S2

A patient may have both an S3 and an S4. When this is the case, the resulting sound is called a "summation gallop."

Like an S3, an S4 is usually thought to be indicative of a _____ ventricle.	Stressed
Also like an S3, an S4 is a very _____ pitched sound.	Low
An S4 immediately precedes _____.	S1
A patient with an S3 and an S4 has a _____.	Summation Gallop

Splitting vs. S3 and S4

How does one tell a split heart sound from an added heart sound? On many occasions, with some difficulty. In both cases, one or more extra syllables have been added to S1S2.

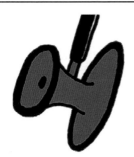

One clue is duration of the sounds. Splitting tends to produce sounds which are very close together, whereas S3 and S4 are usually more distinct.

Another clue are the crispness and pitch of the sound. Split heart sounds tend to be crisp and high-pitched. S3 and S4 tend to be very subtle, low-pitched sounds.

Split heart sounds can generally be heard with the diaphragm. An S3 or S4 can often only be heard with the bell and will disappear if the bell is pushed firmly against the skin. It may also be necessary to have a patient hold exhalation to hear S3 and S4 well.

S3 and S4 are very ___ pitched sounds associated with a ____ heart.	Low, Stressed
S3 and S4 can often only be heard with the ____.	Bell
Pushing the bell down firmly while auscultating an S3 or S4 will usually make the sound _____.	Disappear

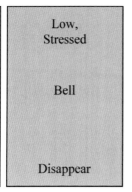

Opening Snap

An **opening snap** is a sound usually associated with a stenotic mitral or tricuspid valve. During diastole, blood begins to fill the atrium, but cannot enter the ventricle due to the stenotic valve. As the atrium continues to fill, eventually the pressure becomes sufficient to force the valve open. The valve pops open, producing a "**snap**."

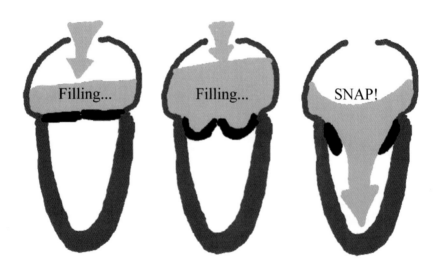

Filling...   Filling...   SNAP!

Opening snaps are associated with ____ of the ____ valves.	Stenosis, AV
Opening snaps occur during ____.	Diastole
A stenotic valve is forced open when the ____ of the blood backed up behind it becomes sufficient.	Pressure

Mid-Systolic Click

A **mid-systolic click** is a sound classically associated with mitral valve prolapse (MVP). In MVP, the mitral valve leaflets are effectively too large. When the ventricle contracts, the valve leaflets "prolapse"; they are pushed back up into the atrium producing a click. Think of the sound a parachute makes when it opens.

Normal Mitral Valve

Mitral Valve Prolapsing into Left Atrium

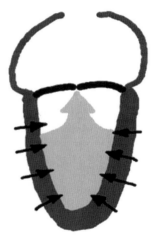 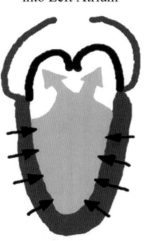

In mitral valve prolapse, the mitral valve is a little too ____.

The valve will prolapse into the atrium during ____.

Sometimes the valve also fails to coapt properly in MVP, causing _____.

Large

Systole

Regurgitation

Pericardial Friction Rub

Normally, the interface between the heart and pericardium is almost frictionless. Inflammation of the pericardium - "pericarditis" - may increase friction between the heart and pericardium, causing a rubbing sound with each heartbeat. The sound of a friction rub seems closer to the surface than a murmur and may change with changes in patient position. It often takes the form of a three-cycle sound, with one cycle during systole and two during diastole:

Rub rubrub...   Rub rubrub...   Rub rubrub...

The rub may diminish for two reasons: either the inflammation is resolving, or an effusion is developing between the heart and pericardium. Use caution—an increasing effusion may lead to cardiac tamponade, a serious emergency.

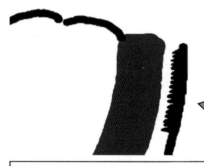

Pericardial Inflammation

Pericardial friction rubs occur when there is _____ in the pericardial sac.	Inflammation
The rub may change with changes in a patient's _____.	Position
Decreasing rub may indicate the development of _____.	Cardiac Tamponade

Hamman's Sign

Most clinicians will probably go their entire career without hearing Hamman's sign, but it is not something that should be missed. Also called "Hamman's crunch," this finding is a crunching or crackling sound that occurs in synchrony with the heartbeat. (Similar sounds heard in synchrony with respiration may indicate air in the chest wall - subcutaneous emphysema—another serious finding.)

Hamman's Sign is indicative of air in the mediastinum (pneumomediastinum) or of air in the pericardium (pneumopericaridum). Both of these conditions signal potentially serious interruptions to the integrity of the airway, lungs or digestive tract and merit prompt investigation.

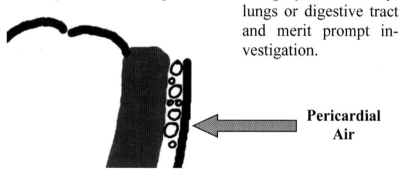

Pericardial Air

Hamman's sign indicates the presence of _____ in the mediastinum or pericardial sac.	Air
This sign usually indicates that air is escaping from the _____ or _____.	Airway, Esophagus

Murmurs: Basic Principles

Murmurs commonly arise from one of two sources: either a valvular abnormality or an abnormal blood flow pathway. Either of these conditions may be congenital or acquired.

Cardiac valvular architecture and function may appear fairly complex but valve pathology can be reduced to fairly simple terms. A valve is fundamentally a door, and there are only a few problems a door can have: it does not open properly, it does not close properly or it neither opens nor closes properly.

Assessment for abnormal blood flow pathways is greatly assisted by a knowledge of fetal circulation patterns and the pathologic conditions commonly associated with myocardial rupture.

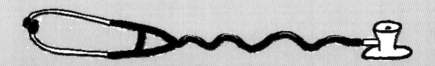

Key Points:

- Four major valves are present in the heart to promote unidirectional flow through its chambers. Damage to one or more of these valves may produce a murmur.

- Valves open and close in response to pressure changes.

- The main things that can go wrong with a valve are failure to open (stenosis) and failure to close (incompetence or regurgitation).

- Blood which takes an abnormal route through the heart or great vessels may cause turbulence and produce a murmur.

- Abnormal blood flow pathways may be congenital or acquired.

Normal Valve Function

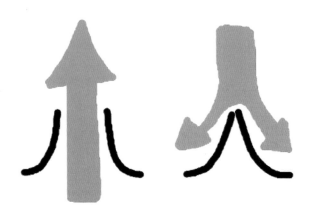

A healthy valve is very pliable; it opens easily, presenting very little resistance to forward blood flow. It also closes – or "**coapts**" – tightly to prevent retrograde blood flow.

A healthy valve presents very little _____ to opening and allowing forward blood flow.	Resistance
A healthy valve also _____ tightly to prevent retrograde blood flow.	Coapts
Looking at the picture above, can you determine which image represents systole?	Trick question—not without knowing which valve this image represents.

Valve Pathology: Stenosis

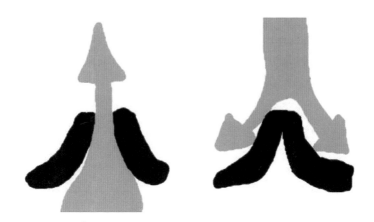

One form of valve pathology is **stenosis**. Stenosis may occur congenitally or may arise from conditions like rheumatic fever or simple wear and tear. This image demonstrates a thickened valve which does not open properly but coapts well.

A stenotic valve is one which does not ____ properly.	Open
As stenosis increases, ____ to forward blood flow increases.	Resistance
Due to the increased workload, a heart chamber which pumps through a stenotic valve often becomes ____.	Hypertrophied (enlarged)

Valve Pathology: Regurgitation

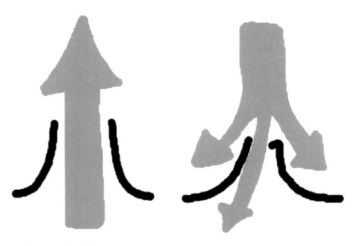

The other chief form of valve malfunction is **regurgitation** (also called **incompetence**). This image demonstrates a valve which has failed to coapt. Among other causes, regurgitation may occur if a papillary muscle or chordae has ruptured or if a valve is damaged from infection (endocarditis).

A regurgitant valve is one which does not _____ properly.	Close
Regurgitation allows _____ blood flow to take place.	Retrograde
Question: Does regurgitation take place during systole or during diastole?	Another trick question—it depends on which valve is regurgitant!

Valve Pathology: Combination

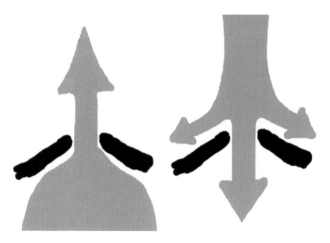

Many diseased valves exhibit a combination of both regurgitation and stenosis. The image above demonstrates a thickened, "stuck" valve which does not open or close well - it is essentially immobile.

A valve which is both stenotic and regurgitant exhibits dysfunction during both _____ and _____ .

Systole, Diastole

A valve which is both regurgitant and incompetent can be thought of as being _____ half-way open.

Stuck

53

Abnormal Blood Flow Pathways

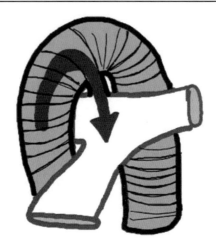

There are a variety of conditions which can cause blood to take an abnormal route through or around the heart. Many of these conditions are congenital. The aorta and pulmonary artery are pictured above. Do you recognize the congenital condition illustrated in this example?

Some abnormal blood flow pathways represent remnants of _____ circulation which did not mature properly.	Fetal
The example of an abnormal pathway pictured above is called a _____.	Patent ductus arteriosus (PDA)
If present, a defect like that pictured above will allow blood to flow from the high pressure _____ circulation into the low pressure _____ circulation.	Systemic, Pulmonic

Abnormal Blood Flow Pathways

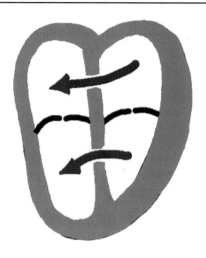

Some sources of abnormal blood flow may be congenital or acquired. **Septal defects**, such as those pictured above, are most commonly congenital but can also develop in a damaged heart.

The image above demonstrates both an _____ and a _____.	Atrial septal defect, Ventricular septal defect
Both of these conditions may occur congenitally, but can also happen if the septum experiences an _____.	Infarction
In most circumstances, you would expect blood to flow from the _____ to the _____ if a patient has one of the conditions pictured above.	Left (high pressure), Right (low pressure)

Describing a Murmur

If you pick up the chart of a patient with a cardiac murmur, odds are that you will see "III/VI SEM" scrawled upon it. On the rare occasions that this description is technically correct, it still omits a great deal of important information.

Describing a murmur takes some thought. Like so many things in medicine, the ability to accurately describe physical examination findings is a great aid in helping you or a consultant to determine what is happening with a patient.

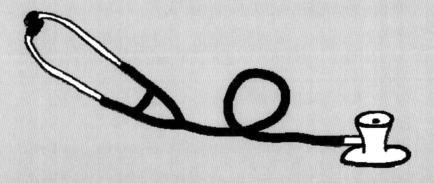

Key Points:

Murmurs are described by the following characteristics:

- Timing
- Intensity
- Location
- Radiation
- Shape
- Pitch
- Quality
- Factors causing variation

A comprehensive description of a cardiac murmur should address most of these characteristics.

Timing

When a murmur is discovered the first, most important thing to determine **timing** - is it a systolic or diastolic murmur? This information is critical in developing a differential diagnosis. This determination may seem elementary, but it can be surprisingly difficult, especially in a tachycardic patient.

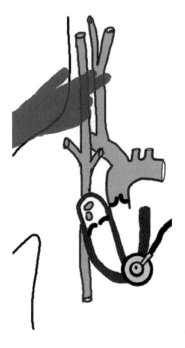

At resting heart rates, diastole is noticeably longer than systole. Since the carotid pulse coincides with systole, one easy way to determine when systole is occurring is to auscultate while simultaneously palpating the carotid pulse. S1 can also be identified as the louder heart sound at the cardiac apex.

As your skills improve, you will refine your ability to describe murmur timing. For example, a systolic murmur may be characterized as early systolic, mid-systolic or late systolic. A murmur which occupies all of systole is referred to as a "holosystolic" or "pansystolic" murmur.

At lower heart rates, diastole is noticeably _____ than systole.	Longer
In a tachycardic heart, systole can be determined by listening while simultaneously _____.	Palpating the carotid pulse

Intensity

Murmur **intensity** is graded on a I-VI scale, with I being barely audible and VI being extremely loud. Murmurs grade IV and greater are associated with a thrill.

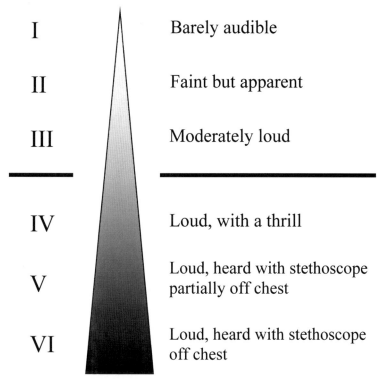

I	Barely audible
II	Faint but apparent
III	Moderately loud
IV	Loud, with a thrill
V	Loud, heard with stethoscope partially off chest
VI	Loud, heard with stethoscope off chest

Murmur intensity is rated on a scale from _____ to _____.

Important to remember: Murmurs with an intensity of IV or greater are associated with a _____.

I, VI

Thrill

Describing a Murmur
Location

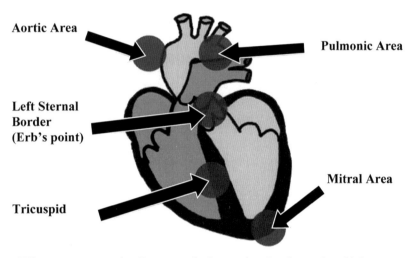

Aortic Area

Pulmonic Area

Left Sternal Border (Erb's point)

Mitral Area

Tricuspid

When a murmur is discovered, the patient's chest should be carefully examined to determine the **location** where the murmur is loudest in intensity. Special attention is paid to the named auscultory locations previously mentioned.

Recall that while most auscultory sites are named for a particular valve, a murmur at that site may be due to pathology unrelated to that valve. For example, a murmur at the "mitral area" may be due to pathology of the mitral valve or the aortic valve.

If mitral valve pathology is suspected, a murmur will likely be heard at the _____.

The pulmonic area does not overlie the pulmonic valve. Instead, it overlies the location where sounds from the pulmonic valve are likely to be _____.

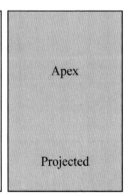

Apex

Projected

Radiation

Turbulent blood flow pro-
duces vibrations which gen-
erate sound. These vibra-
tions are sometimes con-
ducted through the great
vessels to other locations on
the chest or neck. Different
pathologic states are frequently associated with a
fairly typical **radiation** pat-
tern.

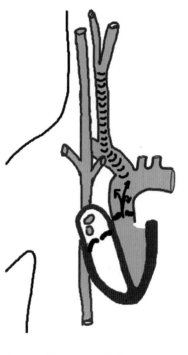

This image demonstrates
aortic stenosis, which causes
turbulent blood flow in the
aorta. If the turbulence is
significant enough, it will
cause sound to be transmitted into the carotid arteries.

Significant turbulence often causes sound to be transmitted to other locations on the chest or neck. This is referred to as _____. For example, conditions which produce turbulence in the aorta may cause radiation to the _____.	Radiation Carotid arteries

Shape

The term "**shape**" is used to refine and further characterize the intensity of a murmur - does it remain constant, increase, or decrease? Murmur shape is often graphically represented as depicted below.

A murmur which starts quietly but grows more intense is referred to as a "**crescendo**" murmur.

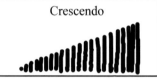
Crescendo

A "**decrescendo**" murmur starts at maximum intensity and then diminishes.

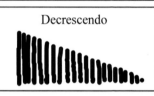
Decrescendo

A "**crescendo-decrescendo**" gets louder and then quieter. These are sometimes also called "diamond shaped" murmurs.

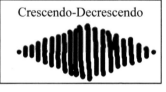
Crescendo-Decrescendo

A "**plateau**" murmur remains constant in intensity.

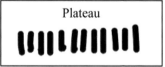
Plateau

A murmur with unchanging intensity is referred to as a _____ murmur.	Plateau
A murmur which starts quietly and then gets progressively louder before concluding is called a _____ murmur.	Crescendo
A murmur which starts at maximal intensity and then gets quieter is called a _____ murmur.	Decrescendo

Pitch

Assessing the **pitch** of a murmur may take a little bit of practice. If a murmur can only be heard with the bell of the stethoscope, it is a low-pitched murmur. Murmurs are typically described as being low, medium or high-pitched.

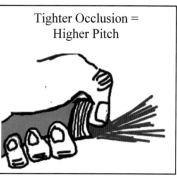

Flowing Freely

All things being equal, a higher pitch usually means a tighter area of stenosis or a higher flow velocity.

As an analogy, consider water running out of a hose. Running freely, it makes little noise. If you begin to occlude the end of the hose with your thumb, the pitch and velocity will gradually increase.

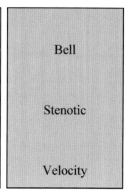

Tighter Occlusion = Higher Pitch

It is very easy to miss low-pitched murmurs if you do not listen with the _____.

A murmur which is becoming increasingly higher in pitch may mean that the affected area is becoming more _____.

Higher pitches are generally associated with increased flow _____.

Bell

Stenotic

Velocity

Quality

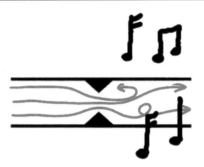

"**Quality**" is a bit of a catch-all term. It allows a clinician to describe any other unique features associated with a murmur. Is the intensity of the murmur constant, or is there beat to beat variability? Does the murmur sound like anything in particular? Murmurs may be described as "harsh," "blowing," "rumbling," or even "musical." You may use any descriptive terminology that fits the situation at hand.

Some murmurs have almost pathognomonic descriptive terms associated with them, such as a "machinery murmur" or a "to and fro" murmur - more on these later.

A murmur's quality describes any ____ features associated with a murmur.	Unique
A murmur that sounds like wind through a tube might be described as "____."	Blowing
A low-pitched murmur that sounds like thunder might be described as "____."	Rumbling

Variation

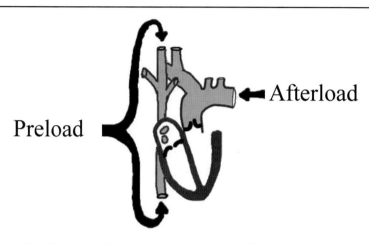

Preload

Afterload

Finally, it should be noted whether there is any **variation** in the murmur related to any actions performed by the patient. For example, does the murmur get louder with inspiration? Is there any change with a valsalva maneuver? Standing or squatting? Isometric exercise?

Each of the factors above alter hemodynamics, changing preload and/or afterload. We will discuss using some of these maneuvers to your advantage in a later chapter.

The work related to amount of blood returning to the heart from the body is referred to as _____.	Preload
The amount of work the heart must perform in pumping into the systemic circuit is referred to as _____.	Afterload
Respiration and some maneuvers can alter hemodynamics and change the _____ of a murmur.	Intensity

Murmurs: Valve by Valve

This chapter presents common valvular pathology (and some related conditions) in a valve by valve fashion.

The goal of this chapter is to demonstrate what is happening at each valve during systole and diastole first in a healthy heart and then in common pathologic states. When this information is mastered, there is no need to memorize the characteristics associated with different murmurs. Instead, you will have developed the ability to arrive at a diagnosis through reason.

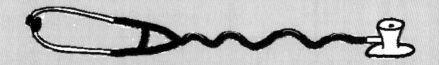

Key Points:

Diastole
- During normal diastole, the AV valves are widely open, and silent filling of the ventricles is taking place.
- The semilunar valves are normally closed.

Systole
- During normal systole, the AV valves close as intraventricular pressure begins to rise.
- The semilunar valves open, and blood is ejected into the great vessels.
- In the absence of pathology, this flow is silent.

Normal Aortic Valve Function

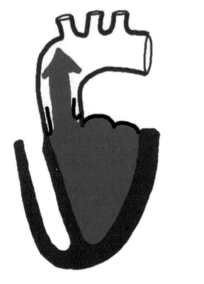 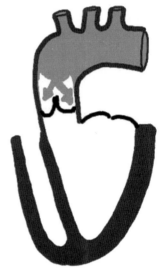

Systole   **Diastole**

We will start out by looking at aortic valve disorders. Normal valve function is depicted above. During systole, the aortic valve usually opens easily and allows quiet forward blood flow from the left ventricle into the aorta. During diastole, the valve coapts tightly, preventing retrograde flow from the aorta into the left ventricle.

The aortic valve is located at the outflow tract of the ____.	Left ventricle
The aortic valve opens during ____ when ventricular pressure exceeds aortic pressure.	Systole
The aortic valve is closed during ____.	Diastole

Aortic Stenosis

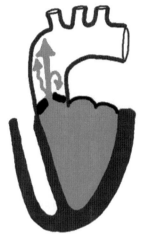

Aortic stenosis is fairly common—if you live long enough, you will likely develop some degree of aortic stenosis.

As we previously noted, stenosis is an obstruction to forward flow. Forward flow takes place across the aortic valve during systole. Aortic stenosis is therefore a systolic murmur.

The murmur will be heard over the valve at the left third intercostal space. The condition causes a high-pressure jet of blood to be directed at the aortic area, so a murmur will be heard there. Finally, sound will also often be conducted in a retrograde fashion to the apex.

The high–pressure jet of blood ejected into the aorta often causes the murmur to radiate to the carotid arteries.

Aortic stenosis causes a murmur to take place during ____.	Systole
The murmur of aortic stenosis is usually loudest over the valve or at the ____.	Aortic area
The murmur of aortic stenosis often radiates to the ____.	Carotid Arteries

Hypertrophic Cardiomyopathy

Hypertrophic cardiomyopathy (HCM) is a somewhat rare genetic condition that presents in a fashion similar to aortic stenosis. It is a good disease to recognize, because it is associated with a high risk of sudden cardiac death.

In HCM, the septum often becomes thickened inferior to the aortic valve. This leads to an obstruction to the ventricular outflow tract similar to that caused by a stenotic valve. Again, since the condition causes an obstruction to forward blood flow, HCM presents with a systolic murmur.

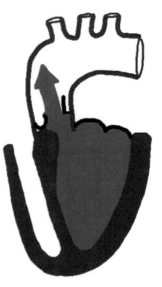

The murmur will be heard at the left third intercostal space. The condition causes a high-pressure jet of blood to be directed at the aortic area, so a murmur will be heard there. Finally, sound will also often be conducted in a retrograde fashion to the apex.

Unlike aortic stenosis, HCM does not usually radiate to the carotids.

Hypertrophic cardiomyopathy is associated with a high risk of ____.	Sudden death
The murmur of HCM is very similar to that of ____.	Aortic stenosis
Because HCM presents an obstruction to blood exiting the left ventricle, the murmur of HCM occurs during ____.	Systole

Aortic Regurgitation

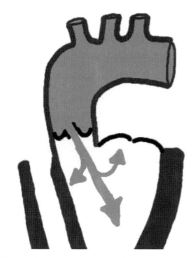

In **aortic regurgitation**, the aortic valve fails to coapt properly when blood in the aorta pushes back against it during diastole. Some blood spills back into the left ventricle, producing a murmur.

The murmur of aortic regurgitation tends to be fairly high-pitched, heard best over the valve. Since the jet of regurgitant blood is directed into the left ventricle, there is also sometimes a rumbling murmur found there (the Austin Flint murmur).

There are a number of other eponymous physical findings associated with aortic regurgitation—they are described later.

Aortic regurgitation takes place during ____.	Diastole
The associated murmur is usually loudest at the ____.	Left third interspace
In aortic regurgitation, a diastole rumble at the apex is called an _____ murmur.	Austin Flint

Normal Mitral Valve Function

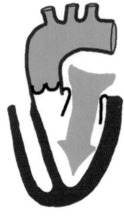

Diastole   **Systole**

As noted previously, mitral valve function is somewhat complex. In addition to having anchoring apparatus, the mitral valve also depends upon proper left ventricular wall function to coapt properly.

The mitral valve is usually open during diastole, allowing blood to quietly flow from the left atrium into the left ventricle. During systole it closes to prevent retrograde blood flow into the left atrium.

The mitral valve is typically closed during ____.	Systole
Blood traverses the mitral valve to enter the ____.	Left ventricle
If the ventricular wall is not functioning properly, the mitral valve may fail to fully ____.	Coapt

Mitral Stenosis

In a normal heart, blood traverses a pliable, wide-open mitral valve during diastole as the left ventricle fills in preparation for systole. **Mitral stenosis** therefore produces a diastolic murmur. Since blood is entering the left ventricle, the murmur is usually loudest at the apex, where left ventricular sounds are best heard.

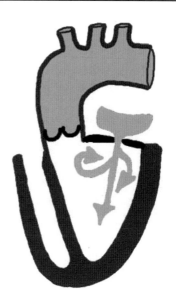

Mitral stenosis is often associated with an extra heart sound called an "opening snap." The left atrium fills with blood during diastole until the atrial pressure overcomes the resistance caused by the stenotic valve. At this point, the valve "snaps" open (see page 44).

The murmur of mitral stenosis is heard during ____.	Diastole
The murmur is usually loudest at the ____.	Apex
Mitral stenosis is associated with an extra heart sound called an ____.	Opening snap

Mitral Regurgitation

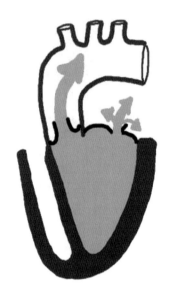

The mitral valve normally coapts tightly at the beginning of systole as intraventricular pressure rises. If it fails to do so, blood will regurgitate into the left atrium during systole.

A number of conditions can lead to **mitral regurgitation**, such as rupture of a chordae or papillary muscle. Ischemia may also cause regurgitation if portions of the left ventricular wall fail to contract properly.

The murmur of mitral regurgitation is heard at the apex during systole. It may be distinguished from the murmur of aortic stenosis by recognizing that it radiates toward the axilla instead of toward the aortic area and carotid arteries.

Mitral regurgitation occurs during _____.	Systole
The murmur is usually loudest at the _____.	Apex
The murmur of mitral regurgitation often radiates toward the _____.	Axilla

Normal Pulmonic Valve Function

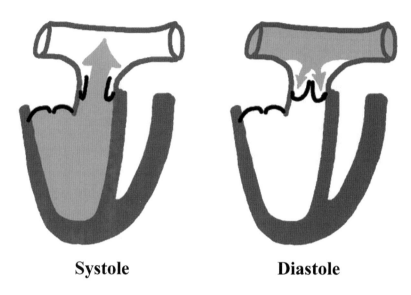

Systole   **Diastole**

The function of the pulmonic valve mirrors the function of the aortic valve. It opens during systole and closes during diastole.

Since the pulmonary circulation operates under lower pressure than the systemic circulation, sounds from the pulmonary valve are more subtle than sounds from the aortic valve.

The pulmonic valve is located at the outflow tract of the ____.	Right ventricle
The pulmonic valve opens during ____ when ventricular pressure exceeds pulmonary artery pressure.	Systole

Pulmonic Stenosis

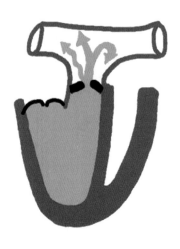

Pulmonic stenosis will produce a systolic murmur heard best at the pulmonic area.

Since the pulmonary circulation operates under lower pressure than the systemic circulation, sounds from the pulmonary valve are more subtle.

One way to distinguish left-sided murmurs from right-sided murmurs is to see if the murmur changes in intensity with respiration. Right-sided heart murmurs generally increase with inspiration due to an increase in the amount of blood returning to the heart during inspiration.

Pulmonic stenosis is also associated with a split S2.

The pulmonic valve is located at the outflow tract of the ____.	Right ventricle
The pulmonic valve opens during ____ when ventricular pressure exceeds pulmonary artery pressure.	Systole

Pulmonic Regurgitation

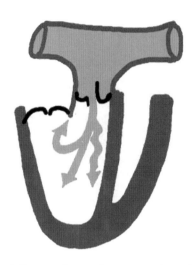

If a pulmonic valve cannot coapt properly, **pulmonic regurgitation** will occur during diastole.

The murmur of pulmonic regurgitation may be heard at the pulmonic area. It is also noted over the right ventricle (along the left sternal border) since this is the chamber that the regurgitant flow is directed into.

Like pulmonic stenosis, the murmur of pulmonary regurgitation will also usually increase with inspiration.

If pulmonic regurgitation occurs in the presence of severe pulmonary hypertension, a high-pitched "Graham-Steell" murmur may be noted.

Pulmonic regurgitation takes place during ____.	Diastole
The murmur of pulmonic stenosis is generally loudest at the ____.	Left sternal border

Normal Tricuspid Valve Function

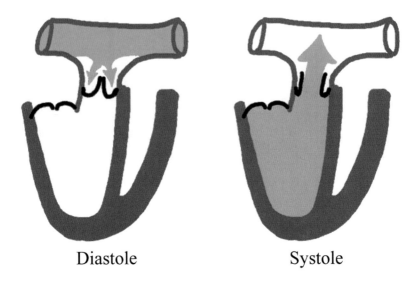

Diastole   Systole

The tricuspid valve normally mirrors the function of the mitral valve. It opens during diastole to allow the right ventricle to fill and coapts during systole to prevent retrograde blood flow.

Again, since the right side of the heart operates under lower pressure than the left side, sounds from the tricuspid valve are more subtle than sounds from the mitral valve.

The pulmonic valve is located at the outflow tract of the ____.	Right ventricle
The pulmonic valve opens during ____ when ventricular pressure exceeds pulmonary artery pressure.	Systole

Tricuspid Stenosis

Tricuspid stenosis produces a diastolic murmur along the left sternal border. Like mitral stenosis, an opening snap may be present.

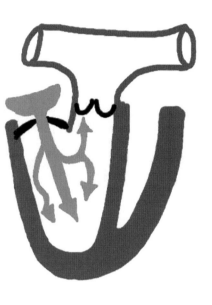

Tricuspid stenosis is commonly associated with signs and symptoms relating to blood "backing up" into the systemic circulation. This leads to conditions like jugular venous distension and peripheral edema. It may be further distinguished from mitral stenosis by listening for a characteristic variation with inspiration and expiration.

Like mitral stenosis, the murmur of tricuspid stenosis may be associated with an _____.	Opening snap
The murmur is usually loudest at the _____.	Left sternal border
Unlike mitral stenosis, the murmur of tricuspid stenosis will usually _____ with inspiration.	Increase

Tricuspid Regurgitation

Tricuspid regurgitation takes place during systole and will produce a high-pitched murmur along the left sternal border.

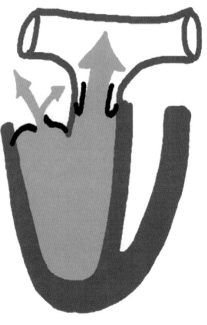

When regurgitation is significant, the pressure is often transmitted in a retrograde fashion into the venous system. Should this occur, prominent jugular venous pulsations may be noted in synchrony with systole. This is one reason why a careful inspection of the neck vessels is a mandatory aspect of the cardiac examination.

The murmur of tricuspid regurgitation occurs during _____.

Systole

The murmur is usually loudest at the _____.

Left sternal border

Tricuspid regurgitation is often associated with visible abnormalities of the _____.

Jugular vein

A Non-Valve Issue: Ventricular Septal Defect

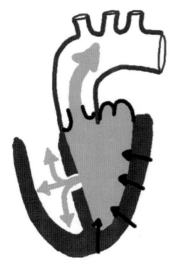

Another source of murmur is a **ventricular septal defect** (VSD). These are most commonly congenital, but may be acquired following a septal infarction.

Since the pressure in the left ventricle is typically higher than the pressure in the right ventricle, systole causes a jet of blood to transit the defect into the right ventricle. A systolic murmur is noted at the left sternal border and the apex.

With years of increased stress, the right ventricle may hypertrophy and right ventricular pressure can increase, causing the murmur to diminish. Pressure in the pulmonary circulation can even eventually exceed the pressure in the left heart, reversing flow. This ominous condition is referred to as Eisenmenger Syndrome.

The murmur of ventricular septal defect occurs during _____.	Systole
Due to pressure gradients, blood usually flows into the _____ ventricle in VSD.	Right
The murmur is usually loudest at the _____.	Left sternal border

Murmurs: Area by Area

This chapter presents pathologic findings as they are usually first encountered: through auscultating a particular location on the chest wall.

Even if a clinician cannot definitively determine the origin of a murmur, it should still be possible to develop an intelligent differential diagnosis for a murmur at a given location. Again, do not attempt to memorize facts in isolation. Turn your efforts toward understanding what is occurring at each auscultory location during systole and diastole.

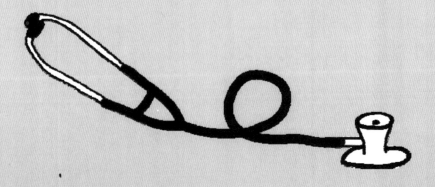

Key Points:

Aortic area
- Systolic Murmur: Aortic stenosis
- Diastolic Murmur: Aortic regurgitation

Pulmonic area
- Systolic Murmur: Pulmonic stenosis
- Diastolic Murmur: Pulmonic regurgitation

Left 3rd Interspace
- Systolic Murmur: Aortic or pulmonic stenosis
- Diastolic Murmur: Aortic or pulmonic regurgitation

Tricuspid Area
- Systolic Murmur: Pulmonic stenosis, tricuspid regurgitation, VSD
- Diastolic Murmur: Pulmonic regurgitation, tricuspid stenosis

Mitral Area
- Systolic Murmur: Aortic stenosis, mitral regurgitation, VSD

Auscultation Areas

Aortic Area: Aortic valve pathology is heard here. Aortic stenosis is heard better than aortic regurgitation.

Pulmonic Area: Pulmonic valve pathology is heard here. Pulmonic stenosis is heard better than pulmonic regurgitation.

Upper Left Sternal Border (Erb's Point): At this point, the stethoscope overlies the semilunar valves. Aortic or pulmonic pathology may be heard here.

Mitral Area (apex): The best location for hearing the left ventricle. Mitral and aortic pathology is heard here. S1 is louder than S2 at the mitral area.

Tricuspid Area (lower left sternal border): Overlies the right ventricle and tricuspid valve. Best site for tricuspid pathology, pulmonic regurgitation and ventricular septal defect.

Aortic Area (Right Second Interspace)

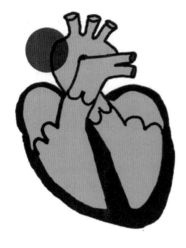

The **aortic area** does not overlie the aortic valve. Instead, it overlies the area where sounds related to aortic pathology are most likely to be projected.

Systole
• Aortic stenosis directs a high-pressure jet of blood at the aortic area and is heard well here. The murmur will also be heard over the valve and at the apex.

Diastole
• Aortic regurgitation directs a high pressure jet away from the aortic area, but the sounds are sometimes transmitted through the blood to this area. The murmur will also be heard over the valve and at the apex.

A harsh, systolic murmur heard best at the aortic area is most likely secondary to ____.	Aortic stenosis
A faint diastolic murmur at the aortic area which is heard better at the upper left sternal border and apex is most likely ____.	Aortic regurgitation

Pulmonic Area

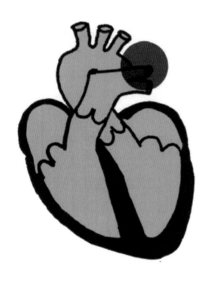

The **pulmonic area** does not overlie the pulmonic valve. Instead, it overlies the area where sounds related to pulmonic pathology are most likely to be projected.

Systole
- Pulmonic stenosis directs a high-pressure jet of blood at the pulmonic area and is heard well here. It may also be heard over the valve itself and over the right ventricle (at the tricuspid area).

Diastole
- Pulmonic regurgitation directs a high pressure jet away from the pulmonic area, but the sounds are often transmitted through the blood to this area. The murmur is also present over the valve and the right ventricle.

A loud systolic murmur heard best at the pulmonic area is most likely ____.	Pulmonic stenosis
A diastolic murmur at the pulmonic area that is also heard at the left sternal border likely indicates____.	Pulmonic regurgitation

Left Third Interspace (Erb's Point)

The **left third and fourth interspaces** are in close proximity to the semilunar valves. This is a good location to listen to S2. A systolic murmur at this location suggests stenosis, and a diastolic murmur suggests regurgitation. If a murmur is noted, the following questions can help distinguish between aortic and pulmonic pathology:

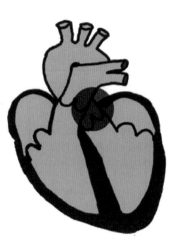

Where else is the murmur heard?
The aortic area and apex suggest aortic pathology; the pulmonic and tricuspid areas suggest pulmonic pathology.

Is there variation with breathing?
Pulmonic murmurs tend to increase with inspiration, while aortic murmurs are generally stable with breathing.

A systolic murmur at Erb's point which radiates to the aortic area is most likely ____.	Aortic stenosis
A diastolic murmur at Erb's Point which radiates to the lower left sternal border likely indicates ____.	Pulmonic regurgitation

Lower Left Sternal Border (Tricuspid Area)

The left lower sternal border is re-ferred to as the **tricuspid area** be-cause it overlies the right ventricle.

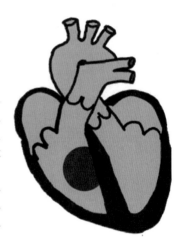

Diastole
- The right ventricle receives blood through the tricuspid valve, so tricuspid stenosis will produce a diastolic murmur at the tricuspid area.
- If the pulmonic valve is regurgi-tant, the right ventricle will re-ceive retrograde blood flow dur-ing diastole.

Systole
- If the pulmonic valve is stenotic, there will be a murmur which is also heard at the sternal border and pulmonic area.
- If the tricuspid valve is regurgitant, there will often be prominent jugular pulsations noted with systole.
- If a ventricular septal defect is present, blood will usually flow from left to right during systole.

A systolic murmur at the tricuspid area that radiates to the pulmonic area is likely ____.	Pulmonic stenosis
A diastolic murmur at Erb's Point which radiates to the lower left sternal border likely indicates ____.	Pulmonic regurgitation

Mitral Area (Apex)

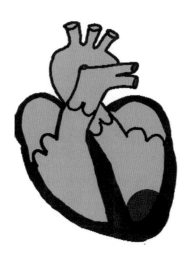

The **cardiac apex** is the primary location for listening to the left ventricle. It is the best site to listen for mitral pathology.

Systole

A systolic murmur at the apex raises three likely possibilities:

- Blood may be exiting through a stenotic aortic valve.
- Blood may be flowing through a regurgitant mitral valve.
- Blood may be traversing a ventricular septal defect.

Diastole

An apical diastolic murmur suggests one of the following:

- Mitral stenosis
- Aortic regurgitation

A diastolic murmur at the apex is most likely ____ or ____.

| Aortic regurgitation, Mitral stenosis |

A systolic murmur at the apex which is also heard at the aortic area is most likely ____.

| Aortic stenosis |

89

Murmurs: Timing

By now, you should hopefully be getting pretty good in your ability to think about a murmur and arrive at a reasonable differential diagnosis.

Another classification scheme that can be used to consider murmurs is determining whether a murmur is a systolic or diastolic murmur.

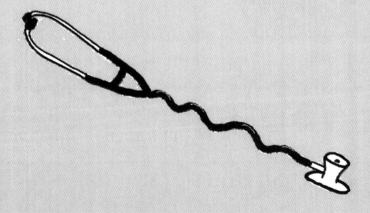

Key Points:

Systolic murmurs may be benign or pathologic. Depending upon its location and radiation, a systolic murmur generally indicates one of these conditions:

- A stenotic semilunar valve.
- A regurgitant atrioventricular valve.
- A ventricular septal defect.
- Hypertrophic cardiomyopathy.

Diastolic murmurs are always pathologic; the heart should be quiet during diastole. Depending upon its location and radiation, a diastolic murmur indicates one of two conditions:

- A stenotic atrioventricular valve.
- A regurgitant semilunar valve.

Systolic Murmurs

This image illustrates the differential diagnosis for a **systolic murmur** heard over the left ventricle (apex):

- **Aortic stenosis**
- **Hypertrophic cardio-myopathy**
- **Mitral regurgitation**
- **Ventricular septal defect**

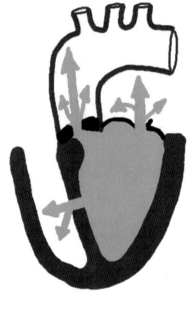

Distinguishing between these conditions requires the clinician to consider where else each murmur is typically heard.

By now, you should be able to piece together a similar picture for the right side of the heart...

The murmur of aortic stenosis should also be heard at the _____.	Aortic area
The murmur of mitral regurgitation typically radiates to the _____.	Axilla
The only systolic murmur that intensifies with a valsalva maneuver is _____.	Hypertrophic cardiomyopathy

Diastolic Murmurs

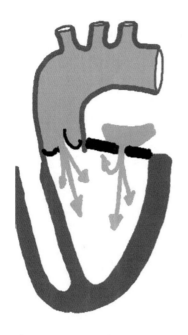

This image illustrates the differential diagnosis of a **diastolic murmur** heard over the left ventricle (apex):

- **Aortic regurgitation**
- **Mitral stenosis**

Again, based upon what you already know, you should be able to suggest ways to distinguish between these two conditions. You should also be able to draw a similar image for the right side of the heart.

A diastolic murmur at the apex is most likely _____ or _____.

A systolic murmur at the apex which is also heard at the aortic area is most likely _____.

Aortic regurgitation, Mitral stenosis

Aortic stenosis

Benign vs. Pathologic

Not all murmurs necessarily herald serious problems. Clinicians dealing with a pediatric population especially need to develop the ability to distinguish benign murmurs from those needing further evaluation.

This section briefly discusses characteristics which help distinguish benign murmurs from those suggesting significant pathology.

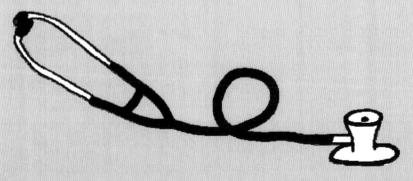

Key Points:

Not all murmurs represent pathologic conditions, but clinicians must recognize those that do. Some important considerations to remember include:

- Diastolic murmurs are pathologic.
- Murmurs associated with a thrill are pathologic.
- The presence of other signs or symptoms of cardiac disease suggests a murmur is pathologic.

Timing

As has been mentioned several times, *isolated diastolic murmurs indicate a pathologic state.* If a murmur is noted during diastole, it typically indicates either regurgitation of a semilunar valve or stenosis of an atrioventricular valve.

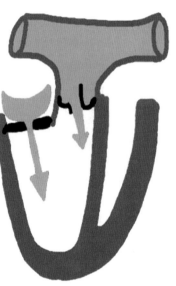

Systolic murmurs may be either benign or pathologic. Further investigation is required to make this determination.

An isolated _____ murmur indicates a pathologic condition.	Diastolic
_____ murmurs may be either pathologic or benign.	Systolic
Diastolic murmurs typically indicate either _____ or _____.	AV stenosis, Semilunar regurgitation

In general, the more in-tense a murmur is, the more likely it is to repre-sent a pathologic state. In-creased intensity usually indicates increased pres-sure gradients and in-creased turbulence.

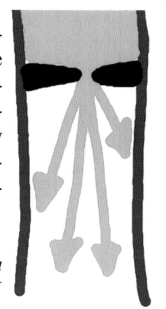

Murmurs associated with a thrill—that is, grades IV, V, and VI—represent a patho-logic condition. Grades I, II and III may be benign functional murmurs or may represent significant pathology.

Increased pressure gradients and increased turbulence will cause murmur intensity to _____.	Increase
A murmur is considered pathologic if it is associated with a _____.	Thrill
Murmurs associated with a thrill are graded _____ in intensity.	IV-VI

Associated Signs and Symptoms

A murmur is likely to be pathologic if there are *any associated signs or symptoms suggesting cardiac pathology.* Most significant structural problems associated with cardiac murmurs will culminate in congestive heart failure (CHF).

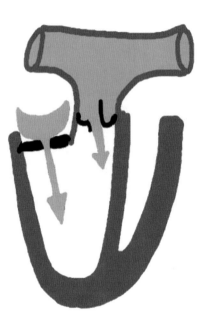

Signs and symptoms of CHF include decreased exercise tolerance, dyspnea and neck vein distention. An apical murmur in the setting of chest pain may suggest left ventricular dysfunction. Murmurs may be associated with cyanosis, usually in children.

Murmurs are considered _____ if they are associated with other signs and symptoms of cardiac disease.	Pathologic
Untreated, most significant structural heart conditions lead to _____.	Congestive heart failure

Common Benign Pediatric Murmurs

Not all turbulence is necessarily pathologic. In particular, the still-developing circulatory systems of children often have areas of turbulence. In some cases, noises called "heart murmurs" in children may not even have their origin in the heart—they arise from turbulent blood flow at bifurcations in the great vessels.

- **Venous hum**: a hum heard around the clavicles. It occurs when a large volume of blood causes the walls of the jugular vein to vibrate. It is heard throughout the cardiac cycle and disappears while supine or with head turning.

- **Supraclavicular arterial bruit**: arises from turbulence of branch points off the aortic arch. Commonly heard above the clavicles and over the lower neck.

- **Still's murmur**: a "twanging string" systolic murmur heard at the apex in children, possibly due to vibrations in the papillary muscles and chordae or turbulence due to narrowing of the outflow tract.

Turbulence commonly arises where large vessels _____.	Bifurcate
Pressure on the ipsilateral jugular vein should cause a _____ to disappear.	Thrill
Still's murmur has a musical quality sometimes described as a _____.	Twanging string

Increased Output

By now, this concept should be clear: aortic stenosis develops when the aortic valve becomes too narrow to allow normal blood flow to occur without turbulence.

What would happen if "too much" blood tried to force its way through a normal aortic valve? Logically, the answer again is turbulence. Therefore, conditions which increase cardiac output may lead to a murmur. Most common among these conditions are:

- Pregnancy
- Anemia
- Hyperthyroidism

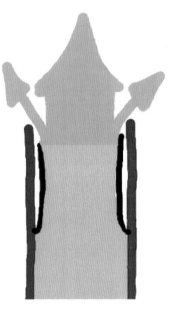

Even a widely patent valve may murmur if too much blood tries to squeeze through.

Benign murmurs may occasionally develop if cardiac output _____.

If too much blood tries to squeeze through a normal sized valve, that valve in essence becomes functionally _____.

Increases

Stenotic

Red Flags

Again, for the sake of review, these findings suggest a murmur or heart sound is pathologic and requires further evaluation:

- Diastolic murmurs
- Murmurs associated with a thrill
- Murmurs associated with other signs or symptoms suggestive of cardiac pathology
- Abnormal splitting of heart sounds
- Murmurs associated with extra heart sounds like clicks or snaps
- New-onset murmurs in the setting of myocardial ischemia or infarction

In most cases, echocardiography can quickly and non-invasively address concerns related to abnormal heart sounds.

A murmur is considered pathologic if it becomes a _____ or greater on the intensity scale.	IV
Murmurs during _____ are always pathologic.	Diastole
_____ is the most valuable test for the rapid evaluation of a murmur.	Echocardiography

Names to Know

Medicine is a profession that appreciates its history and most medical practitioners have a deep respect for medical traditions and history. There is no shortage of eponymous conditions in medicine, and cardiology is no exception.

Knowing the information in this chapter may or may not help you in your hunt to identify potentially pathologic sounds, but it will help you recognize important terms in the history of cardiology (as well as look sharp on rounds).

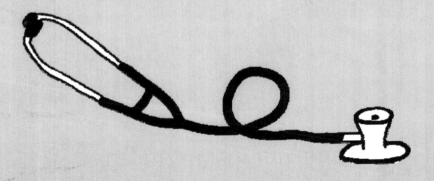

Key Points:

- There are a number of murmurs and physical examination findings named for pioneers in cardiac examination.
- These names will often be discussed in a clinical environment, so some familiarity with a few of them is helpful.

Austin Flint Murmur

Austin Flint (1812-1886) was a distinguished medical educator who lent his name to a murmur associated with severe aortic regurgitation. The mechanism is classically believed to be the result of the jet of regurgitant blood striking the anterior leaflet of the mitral valve, forcing it closed while blood is trying to traverse it.

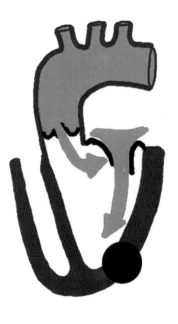

The Austin Flint murmur is a low-pitched, rumbling murmur heard best at the apex.

The Austin Flint murmur is associated with _____.	Aortic regurgitation
Blood returning to the left ventricle strikes the anterior leaflet of the _____.	Mitral valve
This murmur is heard during _____ at the _____.	Diastole, Apex

Graham Steell Murmur

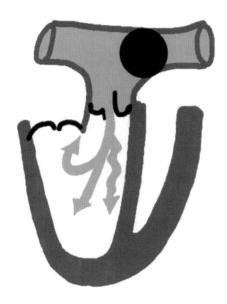

Graham Steell (1851-1942) was a British physician who spent a large portion of his career studying cardiac disease. He was also an early advocate of the value of exercise.

Steell gave his name to a murmur associated with pulmonic regurgitation. The Graham Steell murmur is a high-pitched diastolic murmur heard in the pulmonic area.

It usually develops in the setting of pulmonary hypertension.

The Graham Steell murmur is associated with _____.	Pulmonic regurgitation
This murmur is heard at the pulmonic area during _____.	Diastole

Gallavardin Phenomenon

Louis Gallavardin (1875-1957) was a pioneer in blood pressure measurement and electrocardiography. He recognized two distinct sounds associated with some cases of aortic stenosis. The first sound is harsh and directed at the aortic area. This finding makes sense, since that is the direction the blood flow is oriented.

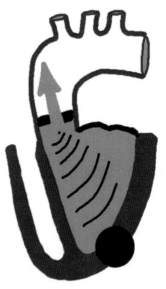

The second sound is a higher-pitched murmur noted at the cardiac apex. This Gallavardin phenomenon represents retrograde condition of sounds waves through the blood into the ventricle.

The Gallavardin murmur is associated with _____.	Aortic stenosis
This murmur is heard during _____ .	Systole
This murmur is typically ____ pitched and located at the_____.	High, Apex

Erb's Point

Wilhelm Erb (1840-1921) was a man of many talents. For starters, this German physician was not a cardiologist but a neurologist. He played a role in having the reflex hammer come into widespread use during the neurologic examination.

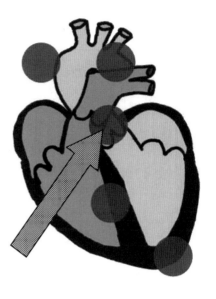

There are two locations named for Erb. One, located above the clavicle, causes arm motion when it is stimulated with electricity. Of more interest to us, Erb also noted that the left third intercostal space was particularly valuable for assessing aortic and pulmonic valve sounds (S2).

Erb's point is located at the left _____ intercostal space.

This location allows a clinician to hear the _____ valves well.

This location is good for listening to the heart sound called _____.

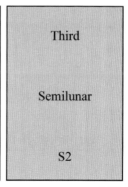

Third

Semilunar

S2

Still's Murmur

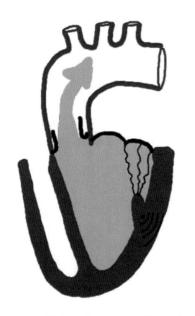

George Still (1868-1941) was an English physician sometimes referred to as "the father of British pediatrics." He described Still's murmur, a benign pediatric murmur usually described as a "twanging" sound noted at the apex during systole.

The etiology of the murmur remains unclear; it is possibly due to vibrations of the chordae and papillary muscles or due to ventricular outflow obstruction. Children with Still's murmur usually appear remarkably healthy.

Still's murmur is a benign murmur of childhood that sounds like a _____.	Twang
This murmur is characteristically heard during _____ at the _____.	Systole, Apex

Machinery Murmur

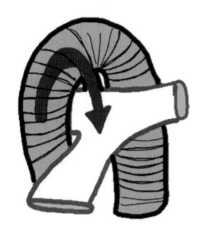

A **machinery murmur** is one that continues through both systole and diastole with a louder and quieter component. It sounds somewhat like a steam engine.

A machinery murmur indicates that blood is continually flowing across a defect during both systole and diastole. *The most common cause is a patent ductus arteriosis* (PDA), a persistent remnant of fetal circulation. A PDA allows blood to continuously flow from the aorta into the pulmonary circulation.

A machinery murmur means abnormal flow is taking place during _____ and _____.	Systole, Diastole
A machinery murmur is classically associated with _____.	Patent ductus arteriosus

Carvallo Sign

Jose Carvallo (1905-1993) noted that right-sided heart murmurs can often be distinguished from left-sided murmurs by taking advantage of hemodynamic changes that occur during respiration.

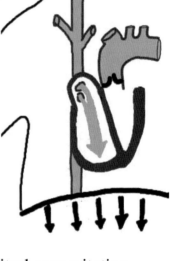

Inspiration causes a greater volume of blood to return to the right heart. This increases the intensity of most right-sided murmur, leaving left-sided murmurs unchanged. Carvallo's sign is particularly valuable for distinguishing tricuspid regurgitation from mitral regurgitation.

During inspiration, venous return to the heart _____.	Increases
This alteration in blood flow will often cause right-sided murmurs to _____.	Increase
This maneuver is particularly good for recognizing _____.	Tricuspid regurgitation

Aortic Regurgitation

While not purely auscultory findings, the whole spectrum of signs associated with aortic regurgitation is worth noting:

- **Corrigan's pulse**: abnormally prominent carotid artery pulsations.
- **DeMusset's sign**: head bobbing with each systole.
- **Duroziez's sign**: systolic and diastolic bruits over the femoral arteries.
- **Muller's sign**: pulsation of the uvula with each systole.
- **Quincke's pulse**: reddening and blanching of the nailbeds with each systole.
- **Traube's sign**: a "pistol shot" pulse heard over the femoral arteries.

Maneuvers

When a subtle murmur appears to be present, or when a diagnosis is unclear, there are several maneuvers that the astute clinician can use to assist in arriving at a diagnosis in cardiac auscultation.

Some maneuvers simply attempt to bring the heart or great vessels slightly closer to the chest wall for improved auscultation. Other maneuvers offer simple, elegant ways to alter preload or afterload to determine the effect that these hemodynamic alterations have on a murmur.

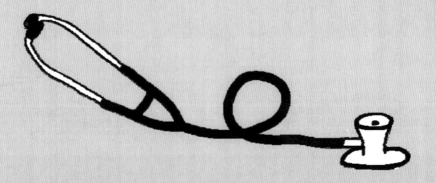

Key Points:

Some maneuvers assist in bringing the heart or great vessels slightly closer to the chest wall to assist in hearing subtle sounds:

- Leaning forward and holding exhalation helps to bring the base of the heart closer to the chest wall.
- Rolling the patient onto their left side helps bring the apex slightly closer to the chest wall.

Other maneuvers temporarily alter a patient's hemodynamics:

- A valsalva maneuver increases intrathoracic pressure and decreases venous return to the heart (preload).
- Squatting temporarily increases preload by forcing blood pooled in the legs to return to the heart.
- Tight handgrasp raises the pressure the heart must pump against (afterload) by raising blood pressure.
- Inspiration increases venous return to the heart.

Patient Positioning

A few simple patient positioning maneuvers may sometimes assist in getting the heart slightly closer to the chest wall. Doing so may make it a little easier to hear indistinct sounds.

If a subtle murmur is suspected at the base (superior aspect) of the heart, it can sometimes be accentuated by having the patient **lean forward and hold exhalation**. Doing so brings the superior aspect of the heart slightly closer to the chest wall. Since the murmurs of aortic regurgitation and pulmonary valve pathology may be subtle, this is a valuable maneuver.

If subtle mitral valve pathology or aortic regurgitation is suspected, the left ventricle can sometimes be heard better by **rolling a patient onto their left side**. This maneuver may bring the apex slightly closer to the chest wall.

Having a patient lean forward and hold exhalation makes it easier to listen to the _____ of the heart.

Rolling a patient onto their left side may improve auscultation of the _____.

Base

Apex/Left ventricle

Increasing Preload

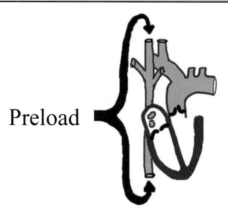

Preload

Increasing the amount of blood returning to the heart increases **"preload."** When preload increases, the amount of blood traversing any stenotic valve increases, and heart chambers become temporarily distended. A common way to increase preload is to **have a patient squat**. If a patient is physically unable to stand and squat, **releasing a valsalva maneuver** has a similar effect.

Increasing the amount of blood returning to the heart increases ____.	Preload
This will cause heart chambers to ____.	Distend
An easy way to increase preload is to have a patient ____.	Squat

Increasing Preload: Aortic Stenosis

We previously noted that the murmurs of aortic stenosis and hypertrophic cardiomyopathy are very similar. Using a maneuver to increase preload can help to make a distinction.

In aortic stenosis, a certain volume of blood is attempting to transit a stenotic valve. If the patient squats, the ventricle will distend, and an even greater volume of blood must transit the valve. This will cause the murmur to become louder.

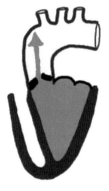
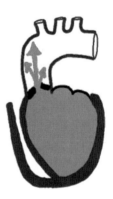

Normal preload   Increased Preload

Increasing preload ____ the amount of blood returning to the heart.	Increases
In turn, this ____ the amount of blood that must traverse a stenotic valve.	Increases
This causes a murmur like aortic stenosis to become ____.	Louder

Increasing Preload: HCM

In hypertrophic cardiomyopathy, squatting has a different effect. The increased volume of blood in the ventricle distends it, and in many cases this actually serves to decrease the obstruction to blood flow. Thus in HCM, squatting will often cause the murmur to diminish. This useful finding helps to distinguish HCM from aortic stenosis.

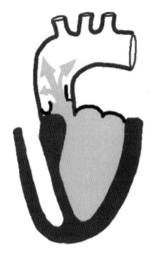 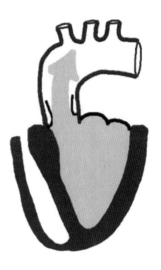

Normal preload   Increased Preload

Increasing the amount of blood in the heart also ____ heart chambers.

In HCM, this may push hypertrophied tissue away from the aorta, ____ the murmur.

Distends

Diminishing

Increasing Preload: MVP

Distention of the left ventricle can also serve to help identify **MVP**. In this case, distending the left ventricle by squatting stretches out the valve and diminishes the degree of prolapse. The typical midsystolic click (and any associated regurgitant murmur) is delayed to later in systole.

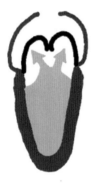

Mitral valve prolapse demonstrating a large prolapse into the left atrium.

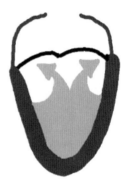

Squatting distends the left ventricle, decreasing the amount of prolapse.

Mitral valve prolapse occurs when the mitral valve leaflets prolapse into the _____.	Left atrium
The hallmark of mitral prolapse is a midsystolic _____.	Click
Squatting distends the ventricle and _____ the click.	Delays

Decreasing Preload: Valsalva

Performing a **valsalva maneuver** raises intrathoracic pressure. An increase in intrathoracic pressure decreases preload by putting pressure on the heart and vena cava, decreasing the amount of blood entering the right atrium.

Decreasing the amount of blood transiting the heart causes most murmurs related to stenosis to diminish. A decreased volume of blood in the left ventricle will increase the murmur of hypertrophic cardiomyopathy, and will make the systolic click of mitral valve prolapse occur earlier.

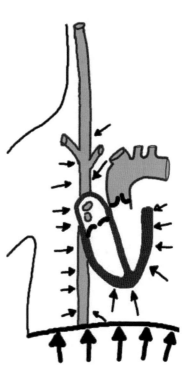

A valsalva maneuver _____ intrathoracic pressure.	Increases
Increased intrathoracic pressure _____ the amount of blood returning to the heart.	Decreases
A valsalva maneuver _____ the murmur of HCM.	Increases

Increasing Afterload: Handgrasp

"**Afterload**" refers to the systemic pressure that the heart must pump against - the higher the pressure, the higher the afterload. Afterload has an effect on pressure gradients across left-sided heart valves. **Sustaining a strong handgrasp** for 20-30 seconds increases afterload.

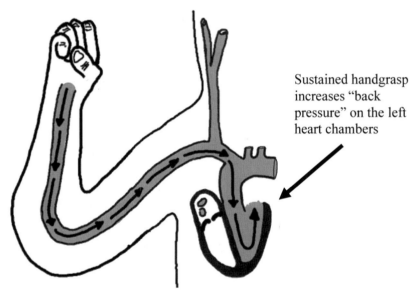

Sustained handgrasp increases "back pressure" on the left heart chambers

The work the heart must do to pump against systemic pressure is referred to as ____.	Afterload
Clenching a fist has the effect of temporarily ____ this workload.	Increasing
Altering this workload alters the ____ across the aortic and mitral valves.	Pressure gradients

Increasing Afterload: Aortic Valve

Increasing back-pressure on the aortic valve
will increase the murmur of aortic regurgitation.

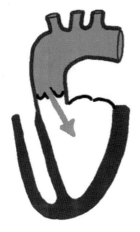 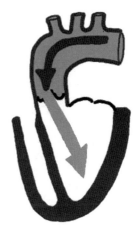

| Murmur with normal systemic afterload | Murmur increased with augmented systemic afterload |

By now, you should also be able to predict the
effect of increased afterload on aortic stenosis.

Increasing the pressure in the aorta will _____ the murmur of aortic regurgitation.	Increase
During systole, increased pressure in the aorta will _____ the pressure gradient across the aortic valve. The murmur of aortic stenosis should therefore _____.	Decrease Decrease

Increasing Afterload: Mitral Valve

The back-pressure exerted by increasing afterload exerts pressure across the aortic valve and into the left ventricle. (Hence the adverse effects on the heart of one form of chronically increased afterload: hypertension.)

Increased afterload inhibits ventricular emptying, leading to ventricular distension. Effects on the left heart are therefore similar to squatting.

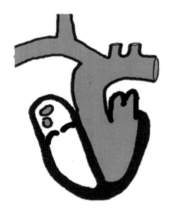

Normal afterload:
High degree of prolapse

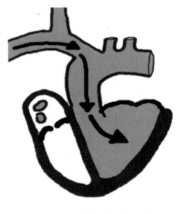

Increased afterload:
The ventricle is distended, decreasing the degree of mitral valve prolapse.

Like squatting, handgrip will usually cause the click of MVP to occur ____ in systole. Given the above fact, one would expect that the murmur of hypertrophic cardiomyopathy will ____ with increased afterload.	Later Diminish

Inspiration

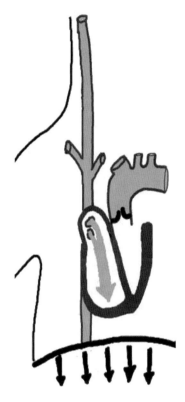

You will recall "Carvallo's sign." Having a patient **inspire deeply while auscultating** is sometimes referred to as "Carvallo's Maneuver."

Inspiration decreases intrathoracic pressure and has the effect of increasing the amount of blood returning to the heart. This distends the right ventricle and tends to increase the intensity of right-sided murmurs (tricuspid regurgitation in particular).

The effect of inspiration on left-sided murmurs can vary. Increasing the amount of blood in the right ventricle can decrease the size of the left ventricle, diminishing left-sided murmurs. In other cases, inspiration has little effect on left-sided murmurs.

Inspiration _____ intrathoracic pressure.	Decreases
This _____ preload.	Increases
Inspiration usually _____ right-sided heart murmurs.	Increases

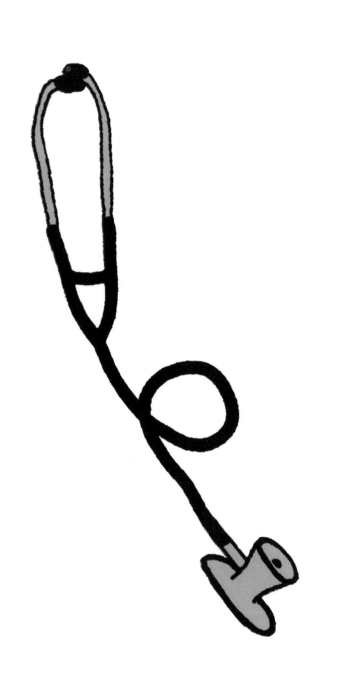

Abbreviations

Medicine just would not be any fun without acronyms. Listed below are some common abbreviations you will encounter (in this book and elsewhere) associated with cardiac auscultation.

AR	Aortic regurgitation
AS	Aortic stenosis
ASD	Atrial septal defect
HCM	Hypertrophic cardiomyopathy
MR	Mitral regurgitation
MS	Mitral stenosis
MVP	Mitral valve prolapse
PDA	Patent ductus arteriosus
PFO	Patent foramen ovale
TOF	Tetralogy of Fallot
TR	Tricuspid regurgitation
TS	Tricuspid stenosis
VSD	Ventricular septal defect

Index

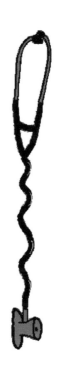

About the Author

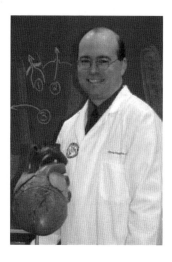

Christopher Hanifin, MSPA, PA-C is on the
faculty of the Department of Physician Assistant at Seton
Hall University, South Orange, NJ. He has written and lec-
tured on topics related to cardiovascular medicine, preven-
tive medicine and health literacy. His clinical background
is in cardiothoracic surgery and emergency medicine.

The author may be contacted at:
Seton Hall University
School of Health and Medical Sciences
400 South Orange Ave
South Orange, NJ 07079

For additional copies of
Heart Sounds: A Cardiac Auscultation Primer
please visit:
http://tinyurl.com/HeartSoundsBook